# TOBACCO, ALCOHOL, AND OTHER DRUGS

Mary Bronson Merki, Ph.D.

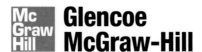
Glencoe
McGraw-Hill

New York, New York    Columbus, Ohio    Chicago, Illinois    Peoria, Illinois    Woodland Hills, California

# Teacher Reviewers

**Susan Giarratano Russell, Ed. D., MSPH, CHES**
Health Education and Communication Consultant
  Office on Smoking and Health, Centers for
  Disease Control and Prevention
Professor, Kinesiology & Health Promotion
  California State University, Fullerton
Fullerton, California

**Linda Salzman**
Health Education Consultant and Trainer
Wilmington, North Carolina

# Credits

## Cover Photograph

Ken Karp

## PHOTOGRAPHS

Corbis: Bob Mitchell, 1; Chris Trotman, 6; Tim Wright, 4.

Custom Medical Stock: 24 (bottom); Siebert, 24 (top).

Getty Images: Zigy Kaluzny, 16; Photodisc, 19; Don Smetzer, 20; Penny Tweedie, 2.

Ken Karp: 23, 37.

Index Stock Imagery: David White, 17.

PhotoEdit: Mary Kate Denny, 9; Michael Newman, 26, 28, 36; Robin L. Sachs, 5; David Young-Wolff, 15, 18.

Stock Boston: Vincent DeWitt, 32; A. Ramey, 10; David Ulmer, 38.

Superstock: 11, 22; Kwame Zikomo, iv, 13.

## ILLUSTRATIONS

The Mazer Corporation: 7.

Jerry Zimmerman: 30.

*Glencoe/McGraw-Hill*

A Division of The **McGraw·Hill** Companies

Send all inquiries to:
Glencoe/McGraw-Hill
21600 Oxnard Street, Suite 500
Woodland Hills, California 91367

ISBN 0-07-826183-X (Student Edition)
ISBN 0-07-826184-8 (Teacher Annotated Edition)

1 2 3 4 5 6 7 8 9   073   06 05 04 03 02

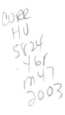

# Contents

Table of Contents

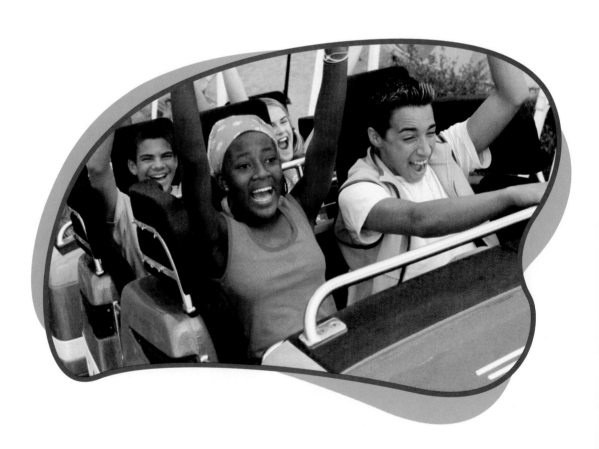

# Teens and Drugs

Everyone likes to feel good and have fun. The good news is that there are lots of healthy ways to "get your kicks." These include playing soccer, shooting hoops, listening to great music, or just "kicking back" with friends.

Teens who use tobacco, alcohol, and other drugs may also be trying to "get their kicks." Their choices, however, are unhealthy ones. The "kicks" they get are too often the kind that hurt. These teens may get *kicked* off the team or *kicked* out of school. Instead, teens can stay healthy, keep their self-respect, and get a *kick out of life* by choosing a drug-free lifestyle.

## What Are Drugs?

**Drugs** are *substances other than food that you take into your body and that change the way your mind and body work.* They can also change your mood and the way you look, act, and think. **Medicines** are *legal drugs used to cure diseases or stop pain.*

However, all drugs—even useful medicines—can be misused or abused. **Misuse** means *taking or using medicine in a way that is not intended.* Forgetting to take your medicine is one way to misuse a drug. Not taking all of your prescription is another misuse. **Abuse** (uh·BYOOS) means *using drugs in ways that are unhealthy or illegal.* Misusing or abusing *any* drug can lead to big trouble, including illness and death.

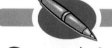
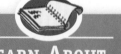

## LEARN ABOUT...

- why some teens turn to tobacco, alcohol, and other drugs.
- the health risks of tobacco, alcohol, and other drugs.
- how drug abuse can affect your self-respect and sense of self-worth.

## VOCABULARY

- drugs
- medicines
- misuse
- abuse
- gateway drugs
- addicted
- overdose (OD)

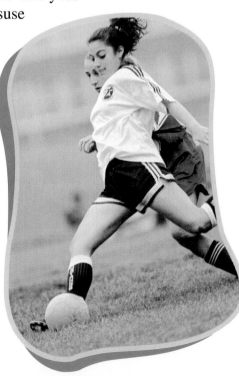

**G**etting your "kicks" from alcohol or other drugs is dangerous. *Name some healthy ways of getting a kick out of life.*

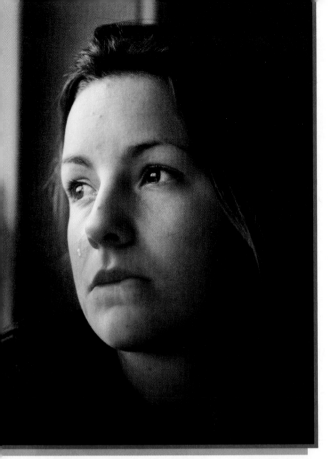

**Y**our self-image is what you see when you look deep inside yourself. *How do drugs affect self-image?*

### Drugs and Teens: Risky Business

Have you ever felt stressed out? Have you ever felt really edgy, uncomfortably shy, or just plain down in the dumps? Everyone has these feelings sometimes and wishes these feelings would just go away. However, some teens use alcohol or other drugs to escape such feelings, to create different ones, or simply to numb themselves altogether. These teens may want to seem more grown up. They may use drugs to fit in, feel more confident, reduce stress, escape loneliness, or battle boredom. There is a catch, however, when a teen starts using a drug to escape a certain feeling, or to get a certain physical or emotional effect. Any use carries risk. Teens are at particular risk, since their bodies and brains are still developing.

## Drugs and Self-Worth

When you look in the mirror, do you respect the person who looks back at you? Teens who have respect for themselves are less likely to use alcohol and other drugs than teens who do not. They work hard, play hard, and stay involved at home and in school. They stand up to their peers when their values are on the line.

Often, it is teens with low self-worth who start using drugs in the first place, thinking that substances will help them feel better about themselves. This plan backfires. Using drugs actually chips away at a person's self-worth. How? The more a person has to lie, cover up, or make excuses because of substance use, the harder it becomes to look oneself straight in the eye.

## FACE THE FACTS: DRUGS HURT TEENS

- Among smokers 12 to 17, 70% already regret the decision they made to smoke.
- 33% of young people who become regular smokers will actually die of causes related to their smoking.
- Teens who begin drinking before age 15 are 4 times more likely to become alcoholics than those who begin drinking at age 21.
- The younger a teen is when he or she is introduced to a drug, the more at risk he or she is for getting into trouble physically and emotionally with these substances.
- Alcohol-related collisions are the leading cause of death for people ages 15 to 24.

## PRACTICING HEALTHFUL BEHAVIORS

### The Power of Self-Worth

Of course, everyone suffers from feelings of low self-worth sometimes. This is because everyone has doubts, makes mistakes, and experiences failures. The key is to be able to put these "lows" in perspective. Learn from them. Look for ways to celebrate your strengths and strengthen your weaknesses. Here are some actions you can take to improve your sense of self-worth:

- **RESET YOUR GOALS.** Set goals that are realistic, reachable, and clear. Always strive for improvement, not perfection.
- **TURN TO FAMILY AND FRIENDS FOR HELP WHEN YOU NEED IT.** Their positive feedback can give you a much-needed lift. Work on accepting compliments when they come your way.
- **GIVE *YOURSELF* SUPPORT.** Celebrate your successes—even the smallest ones. Keep a journal. Keep track of every time you achieve a goal, do an act of kindness, or stick up for the highest values. Use positive self-talk, giving *yourself* a deserved pat on the back.
- **HANG OUT WITH PEOPLE WHO HAVE STRONG VALUES AND HEALTHFUL HABITS.** Positive peer support will keep you on the upswing.
- **MAKE A PERSONAL COMMITMENT TO AVOID THE USE OF TOBACCO, ALCOHOL, AND OTHER DRUGS.** Practice ways to refuse substances *before* they are offered to you. Make a drug-free contract with a close friend and keep it.
- **LEARN NEW SKILLS.** Practice, develop, and share your talents and skills.
- **REACH OUT TO SOMEONE ELSE IN NEED.** There's no better way to feel your own worth than by helping someone else.

## Keep the Gate Shut!

You've probably heard, "What's one cigarette?" or "It's just a beer or a wine cooler." These statements just aren't true. Alcohol, tobacco, and marijuana contain substances that can hurt you *and* can lead to other drug use. The fact is that tobacco, alcohol (including beer and wine), and marijuana are all gateway drugs. These are *drugs that can lead to using other drugs.* Using even a little of any of these drugs can get people addicted, "hooked," or *dependent on that drug.* It also can lead to using or getting addicted to other drugs like cocaine or heroin.

### Dead End

One of the greatest risks associated with drugs is that they can kill. Sometimes, users overdose, or OD, that is, *take more of a drug than the body can stand.* Often, overdoses are unintentional. The user simply doesn't know his or her limit and suffers the consequences. Overdosing can happen with only one use. The person may become unconscious (not able to feel or think) and

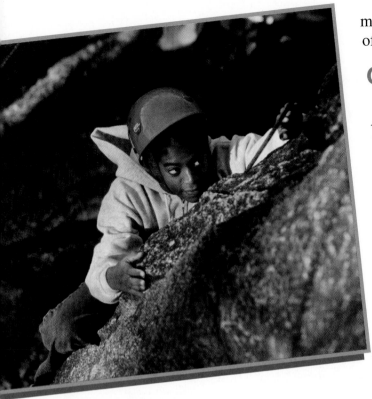

may even die. It is one of the greatest dangers of using or mixing alcohol and other drugs.

## Get a Kick Out of Life

Each year, the National Institute on Drug Abuse (NIDA) does a study on teen drug use. The results of the 2000 study show that, although 27 percent of teens your age have tried some form of drugs, 73 percent of them have not! That means the vast majority of people your age remain drug-free. In fact, more teens are saying no to all kinds of dangerous and unhealthful behaviors. Teens are choosing to get a kick out of life the natural way—without chemicals. So remember these two ideas as you head into your future: when you refuse drugs, you're not alone, *and* you're in good company!

**D**eciding to be drug free will help you reach your goals. *What other positive behaviors can help you to reach your goals?*

## Lesson 1 Review

Using complete sentences, answer the following questions on a sheet of paper.

### Reviewing Terms and Facts

1. **Recall** What are some reasons that teens turn to tobacco, alcohol, and other drugs?
2. **Recall** What are *gateway drugs*? Name three.
3. **Vocabulary** What is *overdosing*? Why is the risk of overdosing so great?

### Thinking Critically

4. **Synthesize** Describe in your own words the relationship between drug use and self-worth.

### Applying Health Skills

5. **Goal Setting** With your classmates, write a pledge in which you promise not to use tobacco, alcohol, and other drugs. Sign it and post it in your room. Remind yourself that making this pledge is one of the ways you can take responsibility for your lifelong health. Discuss with your classmates ways you can support one another in keeping your pledge.

# Substances and Your Growing Body

Tobacco, alcohol, and other drugs are a triple threat. They can hurt your physical, mental/emotional, and social health. This is especially true during the teen years when your body is changing and growing so rapidly. Learning the facts about how substances can harm you will help you make healthy choices.

## How Drugs Affect the Body

The body is made up of many parts. Some of the smallest of these parts are cells. **Cells** are *tiny, complex units that make up all plants and animals.* The toxins in tobacco and other drugs can damage cells. Drugs can also cause the growth of dangerous cancer cells.

Tobacco, alcohol, and other drugs can also damage your organs. These are the collections of cells in your body that work together to perform specific jobs. For example, your lungs, liver, and heart are vital organs that work to keep your body functioning.

### The Lungs: The Body's Airways

The lungs play a vital role by bringing air into the body, sending oxygen to the cells, and eliminating carbon dioxide. Can you imagine the impact on the lungs caused by breathing in poisons such as tar? Tar is a dark, sticky fluid that is made when tobacco burns. It contains many cancer-causing ingredients. Tar gets into the smoker's airways and lungs. It coats and then destroys them. The smoker may begin to have difficulty breathing. This type of condition may lead to lung cancer or other lung diseases.

**T**obacco, alcohol, and other drugs can harm the body in many ways. *What are two of these ways?*

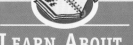

## Quick Write

Describe changes in your classmates and yourself from the end of the last school year to the beginning of this year.

## LEARN ABOUT...

- how tobacco, alcohol, and other drugs can hurt your developing body and brain.
- the damage substances can do to your friendships.
- how the use of drugs can affect your future.

## VOCABULARY

- cells
- cirrhosis
- motor skills
- endurance
- reflexes
- hormones

### The Liver: The Body's Filter

The liver filters the blood of toxins, or poisons. Drinking alcohol can permanently damage the liver. How? The extra calories in alcohol get stored in the liver as fat. Too much fat causes the liver cells to die. This leads to **cirrhosis** (suh·ROH·sis), *destruction of cells and scarring of liver tissues.* This disease can lead to death.

### The Heart: The Body's Pump

The heart pumps blood through the body. Some drugs can cause the heart to pump too fast, too slow, with an irregular beat, or shut down altogether. Certain drugs can lead to heart disease, heart attack, and can even cause the heart to stop with the first use!

## Drugs and Your Growing Body

Tobacco, alcohol, and other drugs can damage anyone's body. A teen's growing body is at particular risk, however. Drugs can rob a developing body of the nutrients it needs to grow. Alcohol and drugs can also slow down physical and emotional development. Teens are also more likely to get hooked, or addicted, more quickly than older age groups.

### Coordination and Control

Your **motor skills** include *control of your muscles and physical coordination.* Alcohol and other drugs can interfere with these skills. They can make simple tasks like writing, speaking, or walking difficult. They may interfere with the time it takes for a person to react and increase the chances that a person will suffer an injury.

### Special Warning for Athletes

Athletes beware! Tobacco, alcohol and other drugs can wreck an athlete's chances of success. These substances can interfere with coordination or may make breathing difficult. Drugs can make an athlete feel clumsy, like a jumble of arms and legs. They can impair aim and speed—bad news for ball players and runners. They can cause muscle twitches and cramping—bad news for swimmers and other athletes. They can reduce oxygen capacity and **endurance** (en·DUR·uhns). This is *the ability to keep your energy level up.* In short, using drugs can threaten any athlete's overall performance and can also get that athlete kicked off the team.

Tobacco, alcohol, and drugs can affect muscles over time. They can reduce muscle strength. They can also impair **reflexes**, *the body's natural muscle reactions.* This can make driving or even riding a bike very dangerous.

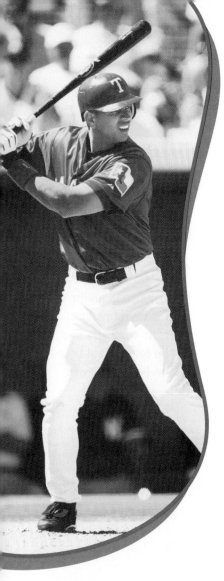

**A**lex Rodriguez actively campaigns against teen drug use. *Locate one of A-Rod's messages, and share your findings with the class.*

### Staying on Schedule

Some drugs can wreak havoc on your body's natural "timetable." For example, marijuana has been shown to affect development during puberty. Other drugs can cause drops in levels of **hormones** (HOR·mohnz). These are *substances in your body that direct certain aspects of growth and development.* Male teens who use drugs may take longer to develop secondary sex characteristics like a deep voice or facial hair. Girls who use drugs may begin to menstruate, or get their periods, later than other girls. If they already have periods, certain drugs can make them irregular. The table on the right lists ways alcohol and drugs can affect development.

## A Developing Problem

**Females**
In females, alcohol and drugs can negatively affect:
- Height
- Weight
- Onset of first menstrual cycle
- Regularity of periods
- Breast development
- Function of ovaries
- Pregnancies and the health of unborn babies

**Males**
In males, alcohol and drugs can negatively affect:
- Height
- Weight
- Male hormone levels
- Testicle size
- Muscle mass and development
- Sperm count and sex drive
- The age at which the voice gets lower
- The age at which body and facial hair increase

## Zapping Your Brainpower

Drugs can also affect a person's ability to learn and think. Teens on drugs have shorter attention spans. They may also have more trouble focusing on tasks, developing interests and talents, and following through on plans and goals. In fact, even when teens who use drugs do set goals, they are far less likely to achieve them than teens who stay drug-free.

## HEALTH SKILLS ACTIVITY

## STRESS MANAGEMENT

### Four Stress-busters

Do you ever feel like you have too much to do and not enough time to do it all? A busy schedule can really stress you out. Here are some things you can try to help you reduce stress and better deal with the demands of your day.

- **BUDGET YOUR TIME.** Use a planner or small notebook to put your day in order. Be sure to allow some time just for relaxing.
- **SLOW DOWN.** Make a conscious effort to do ordinary things—talk, walk, eat— more slowly. When you can, take a break from all schedules. Breathe deeply.
- **TURN OFF ALL SCREENS AND MACHINES.** Enjoy some silence and some quiet time with yourself. The silence will restore you.
- **LEARN TO SAY NO.** Don't become involved in activities that only increase stress. These include using drugs of any kind. Later in this book, you will learn skills for saying no.
- **STAY PHYSICALLY ACTIVE.** Moving your body will help you relieve some of the tensions caused by stress.

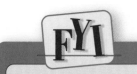

Alcohol and other drugs can zap a person's brainpower by scrambling and blocking messages to the brain. They can actually change the way a person feels, hears, or sees and even make them see and hear things that aren't there. They also mask that inside voice that tells a person to do the right thing. They cloud judgments about what is right or wrong, safe or unsafe, reasonable or really "out in left field." Finally, using alcohol and other drugs can lead to brain damage and even brain death.

## Riding the Roller Coaster

As a teen, you may feel as if you are riding a "roller coaster." Your body is experiencing changes caused by hormones, but hormones also affect your emotions, or feelings. These emotions may seem to come from out of nowhere and to hit you with full force. One day you feel great and confident. The next, you are miserable or unsure of yourself. These changes are natural, normal parts of the teen years.

Adding tobacco, alcohol, or other drugs to this already confusing time in life, however, can make the "roller coaster ride" of early adolescence far more rocky, scary, or downright dangerous. Using substances can distort the way a person sees others and reacts to them. It can make a teen overreact to situations, make unhealthy decisions, or even act out in violent or unsafe ways. In fact, any use of substances increases the chances of getting hurt, hurting someone else, or both.

## Pay Now/Pay Later

Have you ever heard someone called "a ticking time bomb"? Drugs are like a time bomb in the body. Sooner or later, they "blow up" in the face and life of the user. Sometimes the damage happens right away; sometime it is more subtle and takes more time. In either case, damage is done.

For example, short-term, alcohol can make a person fall down, throw up, or pass out. Over time, however, repeated alcohol abuse can lead to problems with the skin, hair, stomach, and sex organs. It can make a person more prone to infections and lead to permanent damage of the liver, heart, nerves, and brain. Overusing alcohol *even once* can lead to death, but alcohol can also kill a person more slowly. Tobacco use in the short term can lead to bad breath and yellowed teeth, but over many years it may cause lung disease and even death. Either way, tobacco, alcohol and other drugs can make you pay now and pay later.

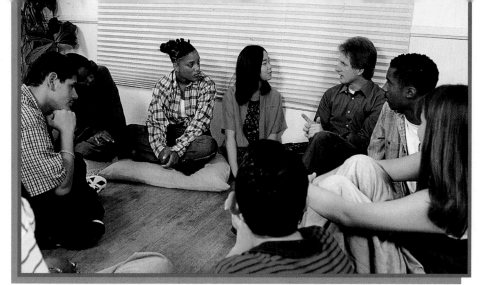

**S**upport and encouragement can help you stay substance free. *What resources can teens with tobacco, alcohol, or other drug problems turn to in your community?*

## Drugs and Social Life

This is a time when you are making new friends at school and on the weekends. You may be interested in forming closer friendships with boys or girls. Alcohol and other drugs can mess up such friendships and make users act in risky and harmful ways.

When "under the influence," teens may act or speak in ways they are sorry for later. They may do embarrassing things, talk too loudly, or act rudely. These teens may do daredevil stunts that they would never try if they were not "high" or drunk. Alcohol and other drugs can wreck how others see a person and how that person sees himself or herself.

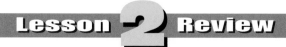

**Lesson 2 Review**

Using complete sentences, answer the following questions on a sheet of paper.

### Reviewing Terms and Facts

1. **Vocabulary** What are *cells*? How can drug use harm the body's cells?
2. **Recall** Why is using drugs especially harmful to teens?
3. **Recall** How can drugs affect friendships?

### Thinking Critically

4. **Analyze** Ian's coach has told Ian that he shows enormous promise on the basketball court. College scouts have come to watch Ian play. What specific risks to Ian's future do drugs pose?

### Applying Health Skills

5. **Advocacy** Make a "What's Happening?" box for your classroom. Look in the newspaper and make phone calls to youth groups and community organizations to get ideas of places for teens to go and things for teens to do that are safe, fun, and substance free. Encourage classmates to use the information in the box. As a class, plan a night or weekend to participate in one of these activities.

LESSON 2: SUBSTANCES AND YOUR GROWING BODY **9**

# Drug Use and the Law

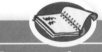

## Quick Write

Describe what you think are the penalties for using tobacco, alcohol, or other drugs during the teen years.

## LEARN ABOUT...

- the laws regarding teens and drugs.
- how you can support your school's rules about drugs.
- how you can show respect for your family's values and rules about drugs.

## VOCABULARY

- probation
- minors
- possess
- sobriety checkpoints
- BAC
- Drug Free Zone

Laws exist to protect you. Laws also exist to protect society at large. Therefore, learning the laws about teens and drugs is very important. When teens practice behaviors that are safe and legal, they are much more likely to lead a healthy, happy life.

## Some Arresting Information

When teens are caught buying cigarettes, drinking alcohol, or using other illegal substances, the law steps in. Teens who break the law can be arrested or spend time in a youth detention center. They or their parents may be fined. The offender can be denied a drivers' license or get a criminal record.

The costs, too, are very high. Besides legal fees and court costs, breaking the law can cost a teen his or her reputation with others. It can also cost that teen his or her self-respect and the trust of parents and friends.

### Laws and Lives

When a teen breaks a drug law, he or she may be taken to the police station, and parents are called. The teen might be sent to a First Offenders program. This program may include counseling and require the teen to perform community service. The teen might be sentenced to probation. This is *a set period of time during which an offender must check in regularly with a court officer.* In serious or repeat offenses involving drugs, there are stiffer penalties. In cases where drug use leads to violent crime, sentences can be long and tough, even for young teens.

## The State of the Law

The laws are very clear regarding substances and minors—*people under the legal age of adult rights and responsibilities.* Selling tobacco products or alcohol to minors is illegal.

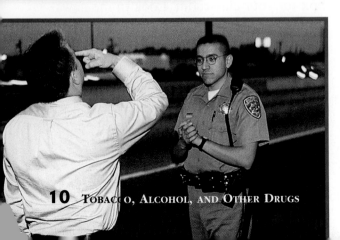

**Using tobacco, alcohol, and other drugs can spell trouble for teens.** *What can happen to a teen who uses these substances?*

### Tobacco Laws

It is against the law to sell cigarettes or other tobacco products to people under age 18. It is estimated that one billion packs of cigarettes are sold each year to underage people. If a person under age 18 is caught buying tobacco products, he or she may have to pay a big fine. The person who sells them to the teen may also be fined.

### Alcohol Laws

If you are under 21, it is illegal to buy alcohol. It is also illegal to possess it—*to have with you or on you.* A teen found with alcoholic beverages might be arrested, fined, and released into a parent or guardian's custody. Repeat offenders get stiffer penalties.

### Drug Laws

Federal and state laws ban the sale and use of dangerous and addictive drugs. Some of these drugs, such as morphine and codeine, are illegal except in certain medical situations. Heroin, LSD, and crack are illegal in all situations. Selling or possession of these drugs is a crime with serious penalties.

### Marijuana Laws

Like the other dangerous drugs mentioned above, marijuana is illegal. The penalties for use and possession vary from state to state. Depending on where a person gets caught and how much marijuana he or she has, a person can receive big fines and extended jail time.

## High Stakes, Bad Breaks

Every year, alcohol-related crashes kill more than 2,000 teen drivers. That's one-third of all deadly crashes involving young people. These crashes also injure more than 130,000 teens.

Drinking or taking other drugs can affect a driver's depth perception (judging how close or far away things are), reaction time, and judgment. It can make it hard for the eyes to follow moving cars. Staying inside the lane and braking can also be a problem.

**What You Can Do at School**

- Stay clean and sober—that is, drug and alcohol free.
- Stay away from peers who bring drugs to school.
- Report drug use to a teacher, principal or, if your school has one, an anonymous tip line.
- Learn and follow your school's policy on tobacco.
- Work with student government or the school paper to make your school's rules clear to everyone.
- Work to get students to sign a "Refuse to Use" pledge.
- Help your school provide substance-free activities.

**A**lcohol and driving don't mix. *How many teens die each year in alcohol-related crashes?*

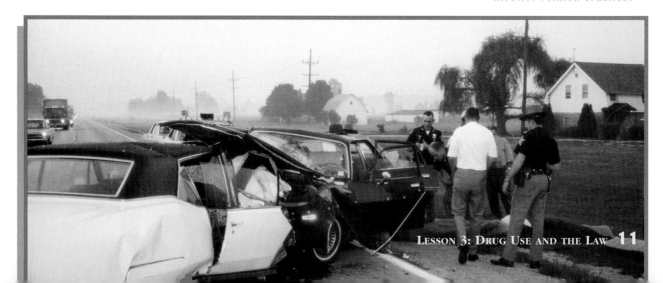

### No License to Kill

Police can stop drivers suspected of being under the influence of alcohol or drugs. Suspects must submit to blood, breath, or urine tests. In some states, any driver who refuses to undergo the test must automatically give up his or her driver's license. Along highways, many states have set up sobriety checkpoints. These are *places where police officers check drivers for drugs and alcohol.* State laws give a clear definition of driving while under the influence. For teens, some states say that it is less than .02 BAC or blood alcohol concentration, *the amount of alcohol in the blood.*

### On the School Front

School rules about tobacco, alcohol, and drug use are getting tougher, too. Some schools conduct locker sweeps to check for drugs, sometimes with drug-sniffing dogs. Most important, many schools are now teaching students about the dangers of drug use and skills to deal with peer pressure.

A Drug-Free Zone is *a 1,000-yard distance around a school.* Anyone of any age caught possessing or dealing illegal substances within one of these school zones faces a lengthy jail term.

## Lesson 3 Review

Using complete sentences, answer the following questions on a sheet of paper.

### Reviewing Terms and Facts

1. **Recall** Summarize the laws relating to teens and drinking.
2. **Explain** What are the penalties a minor might face if caught buying tobacco, alcohol, or other drugs?

### Thinking Critically

3. **Evaluate** Your friend Amy is having a party next weekend when her parents go out of town. She knows someone who is old enough to buy alcohol and she is planning to have beer at the party. Some of the people coming to the party are old enough to drive. How would you explain to her the legal and moral risks she is taking? What other risks may she be taking?

### Applying Health Skills

4. **Advocacy** Research the tobacco, alcohol, and other drug laws in your county and state. Make a brochure informing teens of these laws. Share your brochure with other students in the school.

# Patterns of Drug Use

No one plans to get into trouble with alcohol or other drugs. Still, it happens. When a teen takes that first drink or drug, it can be like standing at the top of a giant slide. The experience may start out feeling like fun. Then, "under the influence" of alcohol or other drugs, the person loses control. He or she starts sliding faster and eventually crashes at the bottom. Getting up from that kind of fall can be extremely difficult. Sometimes it can even be impossible.

## Fads in Use and Abuse

Drug use among teens follows trends. Some years, the "new" popular drug is cocaine. The next, it's Ecstasy. Meanwhile, alcohol, tobacco, and marijuana seem to stay "in fashion" year after year. But despite the popularity of different substances at different times, one thing remains clear: *all* of these drugs damage lives. They can even kill.

Remember this: at any given time, millions of responsible teens are choosing *not* to use alcohol, tobacco, marijuana, or other illegal drugs. Remember that no matter how many movies, songs, TV shows, or drug-using teens suggest that drugs are cool and "everybody's doing them," everybody *isn't*.

## Quick Write

Do you think alcoholism is an "adult" disease? In a short paragraph, explain why or why not.

### LEARN ABOUT...

- the stages of addiction.
- why even one use of a drug can be dangerous.
- where a teen in trouble with alcohol or drugs can go for help.

### VOCABULARY

- addiction
- alcoholism
- tolerance
- withdrawal

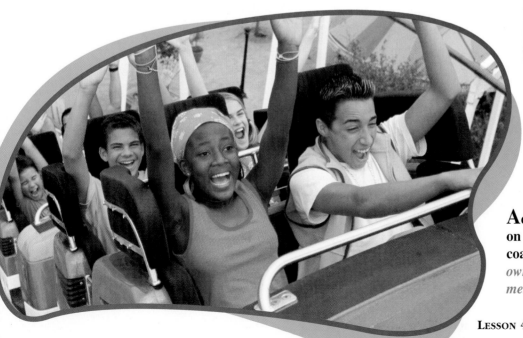

**A**ddiction is like being on an out-of-control roller coaster. *Explain in your own words what this metaphor means.*

## Why Teens Get Started

Teens begin drug use for many different reasons. Some begin smoking because they feel it makes them look "cool" or grown-up. They may be at a party where alcohol is offered. They fear that by refusing, they will look cowardly or be the lone holdout. They think—mistakenly—that using one drug on one particular occasion will not hurt them. Yet, whether on a first use or over time, they will sooner or later show signs of trouble and suffer the negative consequences of their drug use.

### Don't Ask for Trouble

Drugs affect judgment, or one's ability to think and make responsible decisions. Teens using drugs or drinking alcohol are more likely to make unhealthy choices. For example, more than half of teen pregnancies occur when one or both partners have been using alcohol. Sexually transmitted infections, including AIDS, are another risk. So are auto collisions.

Alcohol and other drugs get in the way of healthy relationships. Drug users may physically abuse others. There may be verbal abuse, such as yelling and threats. There may be jealousy or lack of trust that gets out of control. Drugs can create or exaggerate all kinds of negative emotions. Alcohol and drug use also prevents teens from learning social skills needed for developing into mature young adults.

## Addiction: The Disease

Alcohol and drug use too often leads to addiction. **Addiction** (uh·DIK·shuhn) is *a condition in which a person is psychologically or physically dependent on a chemical substance.* It is considered a disease and gets worse over time. The addict can stop the disease from taking over his or her life, however, by getting help and eliminating substance use.

### STAGES OF ADDICTION

1. First use of alcohol or other drug
2. Occasional use of alcohol or other drug
3. Getting into trouble because of alcohol or other drug use
4. More regular use of alcohol or other drugs
5. Increased tolerance
6. Use of many drugs or mixing alcohol and other drugs
7. Total dependency or addiction

Alcoholism is one kind of addiction. Alcoholism (AL·kuh·haw·liz·uhm) is *a physical and mental addiction to alcohol.* Recent research has shown that heredity plays a role in alcoholism. People from families with a history of alcoholism are at greater risk of developing the disease. However, other people can also become alcoholics. Remember that alcoholism is preventable. The secret is simply never taking that first drink.

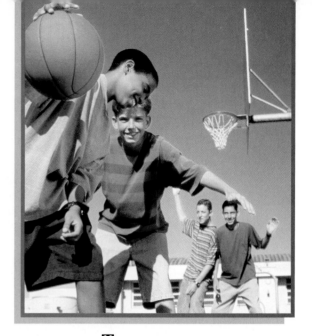

**T**eens who abuse substances may lose interest in school and friends. *What are some other areas of health that alcohol or other drug abuse can affect?*

### The Early Stages of Addiction

The early stages of drug use can "trick" the user. The person who drinks or uses other drugs may think he or she is "getting away" with drug use without suffering major negative consequences. However, drugs "sneak up" on the user, and before he or she knows it, the person may be in the early stages of addiction.

### The Late Stages of Addiction: The Danger Zone

As the addiction progresses, the abuser develops drug tolerance, *the need for more of a substance to get the same effect.* He or she may steal to get more drugs or money to buy those drugs. An alcoholic or addict may begin to lie to cover his or her tracks. Eventually, the drug becomes the central focus of the alcoholic's or addict's life. Family, friends, and work or school are all pushed aside. The person now has a serious, even life-threatening addiction problem.

### The Road to Recovery

The downward slide of addiction destroys many lives. This affects not only the life of the addict, but the person's family and friends as well. Sometimes, however, friends and family confront the addict with his or her problem. They stop making excuses for the user and try to get help for the person's drinking or drug problem. They encourage the person to choose the road to recovery.

Recovery takes time and support from others. At the beginning of recovery, the alcoholic or addict goes through withdrawal. This is *a series of painful physical and mental symptoms associated with recovery from a drug.* In the case of some addictions, withdrawal can be dangerous. As a result, this process is often medically supervised. Once a person's body is free of alcohol or other drugs, that person begins to feel and look better. Recovery requires hard work, but it is more than worth the effort.

**The key to effective counseling is mutual trust.** *What other values could help you to help a friend face his or her addiction?*

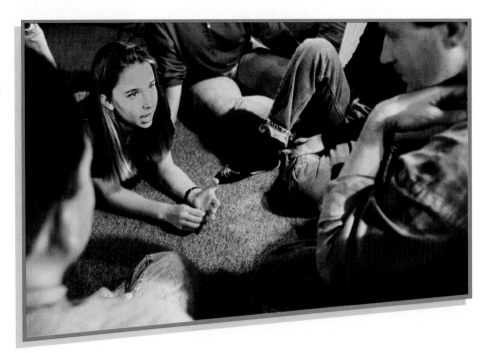

**Help Is a Phone Call Away**

Here are some sources of help for teens in trouble with substances:

- Certified drug and alcohol counselors.
- Trusted teachers, coaches, ministers, priests, rabbis, or mullahs.
- Detox units in hospitals.
- Outpatient treatment centers where teens go for classes, meetings, and counseling.
- Inpatient treatment centers where people reside for days or weeks.
- Support groups like Alcoholics Anonymous and Narcotics Anonymous.

**Family Matters**

When there is a problem in the family, everyone needs help. Alateen is a self-help group for teens whose parents or other close relatives are alcoholics. Al-Anon is a self-help program for adults who live with or are affected by someone else's alcoholism. To find out about Alateen, call your local Al-Anon office. It is listed in the phone book.

## Helping a Friend in Need

A first step toward helping a friend who has an alcohol or drug problem is to go to a professional for guidance. Talk with an adult, teacher, coach, school nurse, clergy person, or other adult you trust. Explain the problem. Don't worry that you are "ratting out" a friend. Maintaining silence is the same as giving your friend permission to continue drinking or using drugs.

Next, sit down with your friend. Tell him or her that you are worried and concerned. Say that you think he or she needs to get help. If you can, have information ready about where he or she can go for help. Assure your friend that the problem will be kept private. Alcohol and drug counselors are bound by confidentiality laws. That means they will not share personal information with others.

# HEALTH SKILLS ACTIVITY

## DECISION MAKING

### Helping Someone in Trouble

Janice is worried. Her friend Sheila has a drinking problem. Janice has seen her drunk more than once. A few weeks ago, Sheila had too much to drink at a party and ended up leaving with some guy she didn't even know. When Janice asked her about it the next day, Sheila couldn't remember what had happened.

Janice wants to tell Sheila's parents, but she's afraid that if she does, Sheila won't be her friend anymore.

### WHAT WOULD YOU DO?

Make a serious comic strip in which Janice thinks through her decision, then tells Sheila what she has done. Apply the six steps of decision making to your comic strip.

1. STATE THE SITUATION.
2. LIST THE OPTIONS.
3. WEIGH THE POSSIBLE OUTCOMES.
4. CONSIDER YOUR VALUES.
5. MAKE A DECISION AND ACT.
6. EVALUATE YOUR DECISION.

## Lesson 4 Review

Using complete sentences, answer the following questions on a sheet of paper.

### Reviewing Terms and Facts

1. **Vocabulary** Define *addiction*.
2. **Recall** Why can just one use of a drug be dangerous?
3. **Recall** Where can a teen in trouble with alcohol or drugs go for help?

### Thinking Critically

4. **Analyze** Teens sometimes drink to feel better about themselves and to feel less shy. What are some other reasons teens may drink? What might you tell a teen to help him or her build self-confidence without the use of alcohol or other drugs?

### Applying Health Skills

5. **Goal Setting** Identify some short-term and long-term goals you have set for yourself, such as college or a career. Explain the effects that alcohol or other drug abuse could have on these plans.

# Lesson 5

# Tobacco

## Quick Write

Describe a tobacco ad you have seen in a magazine. Tell what "message" it communicates about this drug.

## LEARN ABOUT...

- the dangers of using tobacco in any form.
- what tobacco use can do to your health.
- how exposure to tobacco smoke affects nonsmokers and unborn babies.

## VOCABULARY

- smokeless tobacco
- snuff
- insecticides
- nicotine
- stimulant
- tar
- carbon monoxide
- secondhand smoke

Some magazine ads suggest that tobacco makes a person more attractive and popular. The real story, though, is quite different. Smokers can get yellow teeth, stained fingers, and red or itchy eyes. Their hair and clothes smell of smoke. Their breath is stale. These traits are anything *but* attractive or healthful!

## The Different Forms of Tobacco

Tobacco products are made from the dried, heated, and ground-up leaves of the tobacco plant. These leaves may also be treated with chemicals, flavorings, and oils. The most popular form of tobacco is the kind that is smoked. This includes cigarettes, pipes, and cigars.

No matter what form it takes, tobacco can kill. Cigarette smoking has been linked with cancer of the lungs, esophagus, and throat, as well as with heart disease. Pipe and cigar smokers are at risk for mouth sores and cancer of the throat, mouth, and lips.

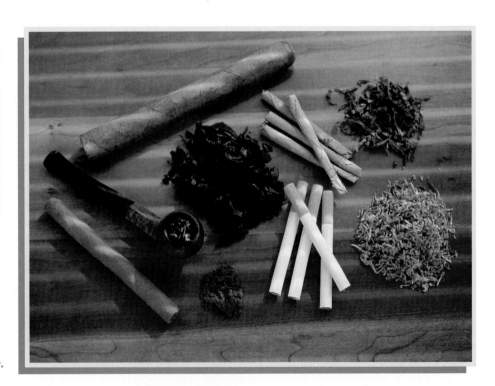

**No matter what form it takes, tobacco can kill.** *Identify one health risk from smoked tobacco and one from chewing tobacco.*

Here are some facts that can really take your breath away:

- Smoking is responsible for more deaths in the United States each year than car crashes, alcohol, cocaine, heroin, AIDS, fires, murders, and suicides combined.
- 33 percent of young people who become regular smokers will die from tobacco-related causes.

- Every 13 seconds, someone in the United States dies from tobacco use.
- Smoking is the single most preventable cause of death, directly responsible for 435,000 deaths in this country each year.

## Smokeless, or Chewing, Tobacco

Some people prefer smokeless tobacco, also known as chewing or spit tobacco. It *is made of dried, ground-up tobacco leaves* and usually comes in a tin. It is either chewed or held between the gum and lower lip or cheek. The excess tobacco juice is spit out. Smokeless tobacco is flavored to improve its taste.

Some people think chewing tobacco is safer than smoking it. Actually, tobacco chewers are just as likely to get addicted to the nicotine as smokers are. Smokeless tobacco can permanently damage one's senses of smell and taste. It can lead to tooth decay and gum disease. Users also swallow more tobacco juice. This can harm the digestive and urinary systems.

Snuff is *processed wet or dry tobacco powder* that is flavored with spices or oils. Like chewing tobacco, a pinch of wet snuff is

## SMOKING: A PACK OF HEALTH RISKS

**Smoking cigarettes has been linked to:**

Smoker's cough

Lots of colds

Dulled taste buds

Bronchitis

Worsened asthma

Emphysema

Mouth, throat, and lung cancer

Strokes

Heart attacks

High blood pressure

Higher "bad" cholesterol

Stomach ulcers

Bladder cancer

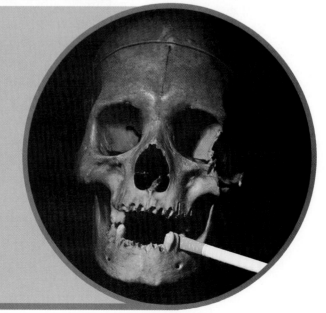

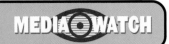

held against the inside of the cheek. Dry snuff may be rubbed on the gums. It, too, can lead to gum disease and cancers of the mouth and tongue.

## The Harmful Effects of Cigarettes

Every day more than 6,000 preteens and teens pick up that first cigarette. Half of these young people become regular smokers. Even when they *want* to quit, they too often can't because they quickly get addicted. This addiction can both last a lifetime *and* cut a life short. According to the Surgeon General of the United States, 90 percent of current adult smokers began smoking as teenagers. Cigarettes are not only addictive, they are also deadly. According to the American Cancer Society, one in five deaths in the United States results from tobacco use.

### Poisons in Each Puff

Did you know that cigarettes contain more than 4,000 chemicals and 200 known poisons? Many of these cause cancer. These chemicals include ammonia, beeswax, and insecticides (in·SEK·tuh·sydz), *chemicals used to kill insects.* Cigarettes also contain the same chemicals found in nail polish remover, embalming fluid, rocket fuel, and rat poison! Why would you want to put these poisons into your body?

### Nicotine

**Nicotine** (NIH·kuh·teen) *is the substance in tobacco that causes its drug effects.* Nicotine is a **stimulant**. This is *a drug that speeds up the heart and breathing rate and raises blood pressure.* Some reports claim that nicotine is as addictive as cocaine and heroin. Users tend to crave more and more of the drug over time. They may smoke up to two packs of cigarettes a day. A few go on to four or more packs. However, don't be fooled into thinking smokeless tobacco can't hurt you with its nicotine content. Spit tobacco has three or four times the nicotine of cigarettes.

### Tar

Cigarettes produce **tar**, *a dark, sticky liquid made when tobacco burns.* The tar is filled with chemicals that can cause breathing difficulties, cancer, and other health problems. New "de-nicotined" cigarettes, which have some of the nicotine removed, contain higher tar levels than other cigarettes. In other words, they are still dangerous.

**To stay healthy as an adult, it is important not to start smoking in your teens.** *What are some of the long-term health risks of smoking?*

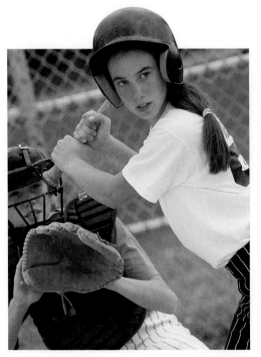

### Carbon Monoxide

When cigarettes burn, they produce carbon monoxide (KAR·buhn muh·NAHK·syd), *a poisonous gas that cannot be seen or smelled.* Once in the lungs and bloodstream, carbon monoxide keeps the blood cells from carrying needed oxygen to the brain.

## Good News, Bad News

News flash! About 1.6 million Americans quit smoking each year. The Center for Disease Control, or CDC, reports that adult cigarette use has reached an all-time low. The bad news is that each day in this country, another 3,000 teens start smoking, and millions of these teens will find themselves hooked on nicotine.

## The Threat to Others

Smoking can harm not only the smoker's health but also the health of others. Secondhand smoke is *smoke that you inhale by being near someone who is smoking.* Secondhand smoke can lead to or worsen ear infections, allergies, breathing problems, and lung and heart disease. Over 50,000 Americans die each year because of exposure to other people's smoke. Frequent exposure to secondhand smoke has also been linked to worsened asthma in children and pneumonia or bronchitis in infants.

### Smoking During Pregnancy

Pregnant women who smoke can do harm to their unborn babies, such as premature birth and low birth weights. These can lead to a lifetime of health problems.

## Lesson 5 Review

Using complete sentences, answer the following questions on a sheet of paper.

### Reviewing Terms and Facts

1. **Vocabulary** What is *smokeless tobacco*? What are some health risks associated with it?
2. **Recall** Name three ingredients of tobacco. Tell what each does to the tobacco user.
3. **Explain** What are some health effects of secondhand smoke?

### Thinking Critically

4. **Analyze** Your older sister, Juanita, is pregnant. She is afraid she can't stop smoking. What might you say to convince her to stop or get help now?

### Applying Health Skills

5. **Analyzing Influences** Find an ad for cigarettes or smokeless tobacco in a magazine. Analyze the message the advertisers are trying to send. Make a poster-sized ad that tells the real story about the effects of smoking on a teen's health. Include the Surgeon General's warning found in the magazine ad.

# Alcohol Abuse

**Quick Write**

Describe some of the effects that alcohol has on the body.

**LEARN ABOUT...**

- what drinking alcohol can do to your physical and mental health.
- what effect drinking can have on your decision-making skills.
- how family and friends are affected by a person's drinking.

**VOCABULARY**

- depressant
- ethanol
- metabolism
- toxic
- dehydration
- binge drinking
- ulcers

You might not think of alcohol as a drug, but it is one. In fact, it is the most widely used and abused drug in the United States. Alcohol is a **depressant**, *a drug that can slow down the activity of the brain and nervous system.* It can ruin the liver. It can lead to serious injuries and death. It can also affect a person's decisions, behavior and moods. In short, it can ruin a person's physical, mental, and social health, just like other dangerous drugs can do.

## Alcohol: The Main Ingredients

All alcoholic drinks contain alcohol, water, flavorings, and minerals. The alcohol found in alcoholic beverages is called **ethanol**, or ethyl alcohol. It is *a type of alcohol that is produced naturally when the sugars from fruits, grains, or vegetables are fermented with yeast.*

### Popular Forms of Alcohol

Alcohol is usually sold in one of three forms: beer, wine, or liquor. Each of these is made from different types of fermented plant sugars. For example, malted barley is used to make beer, grapes or berries to make wine, and barley or corn to make whiskey.

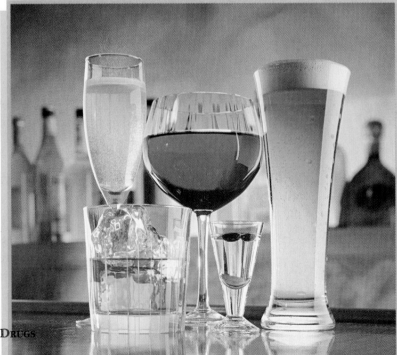

**12 ounces of beer, 5 ounces of wine, and a "shot" (1.5 ounces) of liquor all have the same alcoholic content.** *Ask ten people which of these drinks has the highest alcoholic content. Share your findings with the class.*

### Beer: As "Hard" as Hard Liquor

Some people may think drinking beer is safer than drinking "hard" liquor. They are wrong. The difference is in volume. Yet there is roughly the same amount of alcohol in a standard serving of each. That means a beer, a glass of wine, or a "shot" of hard liquor can all do the same damage. In other words, *any* of these forms of alcohol has the same effects on your body. So if you hear someone say "What's one beer?" or "What's one wine cooler?" remember this: alcohol in *any* form is an invitation to trouble.

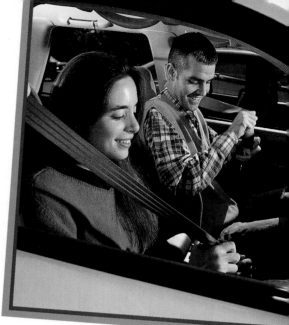

### Running on Empty

Alcohol is a high caloric beverage. The calories in alcohol are "empty" calories, meaning that they don't do much to nourish you. In fact, drinking too much alcohol over time can actually deplete your body of vitamins and nutrients, while adding fat.

## Alcohol's Effects on the Body

The effects of alcohol on the body differ from person to person. They depend on the person's rate of metabolism (muh·TAB·uh·liz·uhm). Metabolism is *the process by which the body turns food into energy.* Once the body has reached its maximum ability to process a quantity of alcohol, any additional alcohol stays in the system. There are no "magic" cures. Drinking coffee or taking a cold shower will not reduce the effects of alcohol. Only time will.

Some of the effects of drinking alcohol happen immediately. Others may take years to develop. Some of the more harmful effects can never be reversed.

### Short-Term Effects

As soon as it is swallowed, alcohol goes to work on both the body and the brain. Exactly how quickly it affects a person, however, depends on a number of factors. These include:

- the person's size, weight, and health.
- how much he or she drinks and in how much time.
- whether he or she has food in the stomach.
- whether the person is male or female.

### The Brain

Alcohol reaches the brain soon after it is swallowed. It immediately slows the brain's activity and the activity of the whole nervous system. With even one drink in the system, thinking clearly becomes difficult. This is because alcohol blocks messages trying to get to

**C**an you imagine trying to steer a car without a steering wheel? That's what it can feel like when you drink. Can you imagine trying to steer your body when its control system stops working? That's what alcohol can do to you. It's important to steer clear of alcohol.

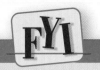

**L**ong-term effects of alcohol use threaten the health of the individual. *In what way do they also threaten the health of society?*

**Healthy liver**

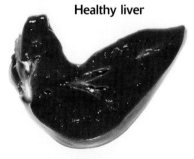

**Diseased liver**

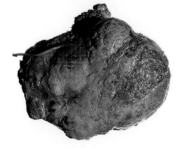

the brain. With several more drinks, it may become difficult to concentrate and remember things. People who have a lot of alcohol in their systems may find it hard to speak clearly or walk a straight line. Blurry vision, dizziness, and loss of balance frequently occur.

Alcohol also reaches the parts of the brain that help a person to make decisions. People who drink often lose control of their emotions and decision-making abilities. This can lead to poor judgment, resulting in unwanted sexual activity, car crashes, arguments and fights, and other dangerous situations. Using alcohol can also lead to depression. Drinking alcohol destroys brain cells. Long-term, heavy drinking can lead to permanent brain damage such as loss of memory and thinking skills.

### The Heart and Blood

Alcohol affects the way the heart pumps blood throughout the body. Drinking a lot of alcohol can lead to high blood pressure, heart attack, and stroke. All of these conditions are life threatening.

Alcohol widens the blood vessels, bringing the blood closer to the surface of the skin. The drinker feels warm, although his or her temperature may be dropping.

### The Liver and Kidneys

The liver filters alcohol from the bloodstream and takes it out of the body. The liver is able to process about half an ounce of alcohol per hour. Beyond this, the body experiences toxic—or *poisoning*—effects from the alcohol.

Alcohol causes the kidneys to make more urine. This can lead to dehydration (dee·hy·DRAY·shuhn), *the loss of important body fluids.* This is the reason why people who drink too much feel thirsty the next day.

### Die-Hards

Even first-time drinkers can die from alcohol. A teen might start out in a supposedly "fun" event. This may be a dare to drink a lot of alcohol as quickly as possible. This is called binge drinking. Binge drinking is *drinking four or five or more drinks in a short period of time.* It is very dangerous because too much alcohol in a short time span can cause the person's nervous system to slow down dramatically. It can also cause irregular heartbeat. It can even cause breathing to stop. Any of these can lead to death. Sometimes binge drinkers even choke to death on their own vomit.

# Long-Term Effects

Drinking over time can lead to major health problems and even death. Some 32 percent of deaths among American teens are related to heavy alcohol use. Long-term use can lead to vitamin deficiencies, sexual problems, and other serious conditions in the body and brain.

Too much alcohol over time can destroy liver tissue. Because the liver cannot perform its work, the person may develop high blood pressure. In time, cirrhosis occurs. Symptoms include bleeding, swelling, infections, and a yellowish appearance. Cirrhosis cannot be reversed and can lead to death. One in five heavy drinkers develops cirrhosis.

Large amounts of alcohol can irritate the lining of the stomach. This can lead to **ulcers**, *open sores in the stomach lining.* Heavy drinking can also lead to muscle and bone weakness, kidney damage, and cancers of the mouth and pancreas.

# Putting Others at Risk

When a pregnant woman drinks alcohol, it can travel along the bloodstream through the umbilical cord. This is the tube that delivers blood and oxygen to the unborn baby. The baby is placed at risk for *fetal alcohol syndrome (FAS).* An FAS baby may have birth defects such as a small head and a small brain. As these babies grow, they may suffer from speech problems, limited attention span, and severe learning disabilities.

## Lesson 6 Review

Using complete sentences, answer the following questions on a sheet of paper.

### Reviewing Terms and Facts

1. **Recall** List some short-term effects of using alcohol.
2. **Recall** What kinds of long-term damage can alcohol do to a person?

### Thinking Critically

3. **Analyze** You are at a party and someone challenges your friend to a drinking contest. You try to convince him not to do it and he says, "Give me three reasons." How would you respond?

### Applying Health Skills

4. **Advocacy** Alcohol companies frequently advertise their products on tee shirts. Design an anti-drinking tee shirt. Using the short-term and long-term risk information, create a catchy anti-drinking slogan and message. Add other facts to make your tee shirt a good marketing tool against drinking.

# Marijuana, Inhalants, and Steroids

**LEARN ABOUT...**

- the dangers of using marijuana.
- how inhalants harm the body.
- the effects of anabolic steroids on the body.

**VOCABULARY**

- marijuana
- hallucinogen
- paranoia
- inhalants
- anabolic steroids

Most teens know that using drugs like crack or heroin can mean big trouble. Too often, though, some teens think smoking marijuana, sniffing glue, or taking steroids is harmless. They are wrong—sometimes dead wrong. *All* of these substances are harmful. Besides being dangerous, abusing these substances is also illegal.

## Marijuana

**Marijuana** (mar·uh·WAHN·uh) is *made from the dried leaves and flowers of the hemp plant, cannabis.* It is the most widely used illegal drug. It is often the first drug teens turn to after alcohol. Marijuana is also known as pot, weed, or grass.

### Effects of Marijuana

Marijuana can have different effects on different users. It can act as a stimulant or a depressant. For most users, it is a **hallucinogen** (huh·LOO·sin·uh·jen). This is *a drug that creates imaginary images or distorts real ones in the user's mind.* The user may see and hear things that are not really there. The immediate effects of a marijuana high include feeling relaxed, talkative, or giddy. The user may have trouble remembering what was just done or said. He or she may chatter on, making no sense. The person's eyes can get red and bloodshot, and he or she may have trouble walking. Some users feel confused, shaky, or panicky. Others experience **paranoia**, *a feeling that others are out to get them.*

**D**rugs such as marijuana can make you see things in a distorted, mixed-up way. *What are some other dangers of using this drug?*

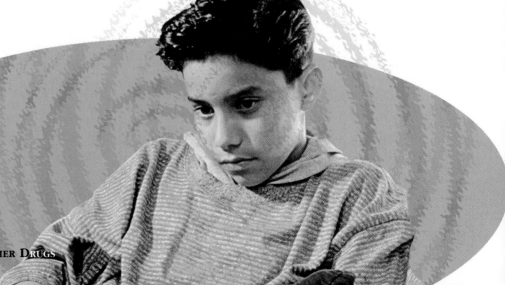

## BODY SLAMS

Using marijuana can harm the body in a number of ways:

- Heart rate can increase to dangerous levels.
- Smoke can damage the respiratory system, especially the lungs.
- Motor skills can be affected for hours.
- User can experience panic attacks—feelings of terror accompanied by sweating and trembling.
- Long-term use can make the user lose motivation and ambition.
- Long-term use can damage the reproductive system.
- Long-term use may reduce the body's immune system, making user more likely to catch infections.

### THC—Not for Me

The main mind-altering chemical in marijuana is delta-9 tetrahydrocannabinol, or THC. THC impairs coordination, judgment, and sense perception. Even with small doses, these effects can last up to 48 hours—long after the "high" feeling goes away. THC is stored in the body's fat. Traces of it can remain present in the blood for as long as a month. Urine or hair tests can show its presence weeks after use.

### Risking Your Future

As with tobacco, smoking marijuana can worsen breathing problems like asthma. Regular use can damage the lungs. This damage can be more severe than in cigarette use because marijuana smoke is usually inhaled deeply and held in for a while. In fact, marijuana contains more of certain cancer-causing chemicals than tobacco does.

In males, smoking marijuana has been shown to reduce the level of testosterone, a key male hormone, as well as damaging the sperm. Using the drug often can actually cause a male to become sterile, or unable to have children.

Frequent marijuana use may cause females to have irregular periods. For women who are pregnant, smoking marijuana may increase their chances of a miscarriage. When a pregnant female smokes marijuana, she risks lasting damage to her unborn baby. One possible consequence is Fetal Marijuana Syndrome, which causes babies to have low birth weights and problems developing normally.

**A Deadly Mix**
Marijuana may be mixed with anything from grass clippings to PCP, also called *angel dust.* On the street, marijuana plus PCP is called "super grass" or "killer weed." Marijuana mixed with opium is known as "O.J." Marijuana mixed with heroin is known as "atom bomb" or "A-bomb." Without the user's knowing it, marijuana may even be mixed with a horse tranquilizer or embalming fluid. Whatever you call it, marijuana plus hidden add-ons can be a deadly mix.

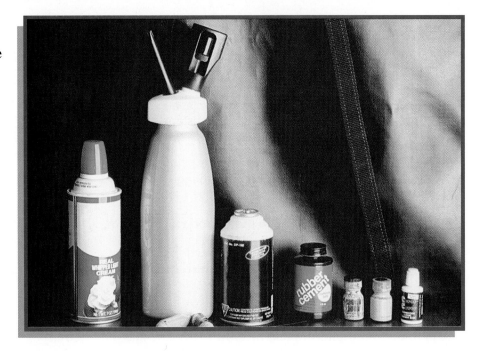

### Road to Nowhere

Research has shown that people who smoke marijuana regularly for a prolonged period of time can experience changes in the personality and the brain. They tend to lose ambition, motivation, and concern for the future. They have trouble learning and remembering. Often, others lose interest in them, too.

## Inhalants

**Inhalants** (in·HAY·luhnts) are *the vapors of chemicals that are sniffed or inhaled to get a "high."* Most inhalants are household products that are not meant to be taken into the body. Many contain dangerous poisons whose fumes should be avoided and *never* intentionally inhaled.

Inhalant use is a problem primarily among preteens and teens—the typical user starts at about age 12. In fact, among younger teens, inhalants are as popular as marijuana. One in five students will have used inhalants before reaching the eighth grade.

Using inhalants can cause death the very first time a person uses an inhalant. Users who breathe inhalants out of plastic bags have also suffocated and choked to death. Inhalants can cause permanent damage to the liver, kidneys, and brain. They can harm bone marrow, which creates the body's blood cells. Inhalants have also been linked to leukemia, a sometimes fatal form of cancer. A teen who experiments with any inhalant even once is taking a *deadly* risk.

# Anabolic Steroids

**Anabolic steroids** (a·nuh·BAH·lik STEHR·oydz) are *synthetic (human-made) forms of the male hormone testosterone.* As a medicine, steroids are prescribed for patients who have diseases that weaken muscles. They are also sometimes used in treating burns, bone diseases, and cancer. These are legal uses.

When used illegally, as they are by some athletes, steroids can do serious bodily harm. They can also negatively affect a teen's future. Athletes caught using steroids are usually kicked off the team. They may be expelled from school. The long-term costs to a person's physical and mental health are not worth the price of any title or win—especially a dishonest, drug-enhanced win.

### Losing by Gaining

Teens who use steroids want to "bulk up"—gain weight and develop big muscles. Other parts of their body end up paying the price. In male teens, steroids may cause the testicles to shrink. The drugs may stunt the body's overall growth. In females, steroids can affect the production of estrogen, an important female hormone. This leads to a masculine-looking body, deeper voice, and facial hair. In both males and females, steroid use can damage the liver and kidneys and increase the risk of heart disease, high blood pressure, and strokes, cancer, and sterility. Steroids can also cause severe acne and hair loss or thinning in both males and females.

**"Roid" Rage**
Frequently, people who abuse steroids become more aggressive. Violent blowups can occur in which users lose all control. They may destroy property, attack other people, or harm themselves—things they would never do in a drug-free condition.

## Lesson 7 Review

Using complete sentences, answer the following questions on a sheet of paper.

### Reviewing Terms and Facts

1. **Vocabulary** Define *inhalants*. What are the dangers of using these substances?
2. **Recall** Summarize some of the effects that anabolic steroids have on the body.

### Thinking Critically

3. **Synthesize** Describe the relationship between violence and the three kinds of drugs you have just read about.

### Applying Health Skills

4. **Advocacy** Investigate the effects of marijuana on drivers. Using the information you gather, write a short play about a teen who, out of concern for his own and others' safety, refuses to ride in a car driven by a teen who was high on marijuana the day before. Read the script out loud with a partner.

# Other Illegal Drugs

Quick Write

Write a short paragraph describing three facts that you have heard or read about drugs such as cocaine, LSD, or Ecstasy.

LEARN ABOUT...

- the effects of stimulants and depressants.
- the dangers of various club drugs.
- the risks of using narcotics and hallucinogens like PCP.

VOCABULARY

- stimulants
- crack
- club drugs
- depressants
- tranquilizers
- narcotics
- heroin
- PCP
- LSD

Taking drugs is like walking a tightrope without a safety net. A teen who uses drugs may feel at first like he or she is flying high, but the feeling won't last. There will be a fall. The person will "crash," or come down from that high. There are many different kinds of drugs that can cause such problems and effects. It is important to know their names—regular and *slang.* It is even more important to know the effects they cause and to realize that the result of using *any* of these drugs can be serious, lasting, and even deadly.

## Stimulants

**Stimulants** (STIM·yuh·luhnts) are *drugs that speed up the nervous system.* Stimulants make the heart pump harder and speed up breathing. Stimulants seem to give the user endless energy and uncontrolled power. However, they really put the body into a state of emergency, the way you might feel if you looked up and saw a car about to hit you. That sudden "emergency energy" or "rush" is what stimulants produce. The body and brain can become addicted to and exhausted by that rush.

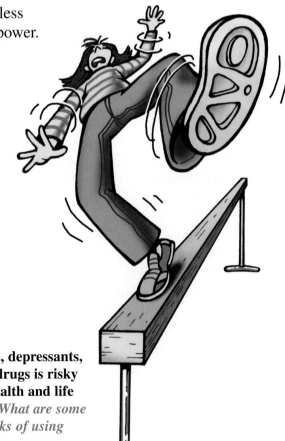

**U**sing stimulants, depressants, or other serious drugs is risky business. Your health and life may be at stake. *What are some specific health risks of using these substances?*

## Amphetamines: Speed Demons

Among the most widely abused stimulants is a class of drugs called *amphetamines* (am·FEH·tuh·meenz). Nicknamed *speed,* amphetamines do just that—speed up the body's systems. As the "high" wears off, the user may experience a severe letdown. Users can also become overstimulated, needing a tranquilizer to calm down. This up-and-down cycle can lead to addiction. Amphetamines can also cause panic attacks, mood swings, sleeplessness, diarrhea, a foul taste in the mouth, dental problems, fainting, sweating, high fevers, coma, and death.

## Cocaine

Cocaine is a white powder made from the leaves of the coca plant. Its nicknames include *snow* and *coke.* Cocaine can make a person feel either "edgy" or deeply depressed. The drug causes increases in blood pressure, heart rate, breathing rate, and body temperature. It can cause paranoia and brain seizures, and reduce the body's ability to fight infection. Cocaine is sniffed, snorted, smoked, or injected by needle. Shared needles can lead to hepatitis or HIV/AIDS.

## Crack

An especially dangerous form of cocaine is **crack**. This is *a crystallized form of cocaine that can be smoked.* Also known as *rock* or *freebase,* crack is made by heating cocaine with ammonia or baking soda and water. Crack reaches the brain within seconds of being smoked or injected. Many users get addicted to crack the first time they try it. Smoking crack can also cause permanent lung damage.

At first, cocaine and crack may give a "rush," that temporary feeling of being high, excited, or alert. The user may feel no need for food or sleep for long periods. Then comes the "crash." This crash can be so painful or uncomfortable that the user looks for more of the drug. Cocaine and crack can cause sudden, fatal heart attacks, even in first-time users.

## Crank

Another very potent amphetamine is methamphetamine, or *crank.* In recent years, the drug has gained popularity as a club drug. **Club drugs** are *illegal substances that got their start at adult dance clubs.* Their use is now becoming more widespread at teen parties.

Most methamphetamine is homemade. It is a coarse powder, crystal, or chunks (*ice* or *glass*). Crank can be smoked, swallowed,

**Diet Pill Dangers**
Sometimes people use amphetamines to control their appetite in an attempt to lose weight. Relying on a drug to lose weight can lead to serious health problems, including addiction. The best way to maintain a healthy weight is through a nutritious eating plan and regular physical activity.

or snorted. The user can get an intense rush. This feeling lasts only a few minutes; then negative effects take over. These include terrifying hallucinations, violent behavior, and trouble sleeping. Often, just the fumes alone can be deadly. Using this drug can also lead to convulsions and brain damage.

## Depressants

**Depressants** (dih·PREH·suhnts) are *drugs that slow down the nervous system.* Alcohol, discussed in Lesson 6, is a depressant drug. Sometimes called "downers," depressants give a relaxed or sleepy feeling. Later, however, depressants can interfere with movement, thought, and action. They can slow down the breathing and heart rate so much that a person is at risk of dying.

### Roofies (Rohypnol)

One of the strongest depressants currently available is Rohypnol. This club drug causes blackout, drowsiness, dizziness, and memory loss. Nicknamed *roofies* or *the forget pill,* the drug has been involved in a particularly ugly, vicious crime. When slipped into the drink of an unsuspecting person, it can cause unconsciousness, and the victim can be sexually assaulted. The victim can awaken with no memory of what happened. It is a serious crime to use such drugs to commit rape.

### Grievous Bodily Harm (GHB)

GHB is another club drug that has made the news. Like Rohypnol, it has been involved in date rapes. It is also odorless and colorless and can be slipped into someone's drink without detection. It has also been responsible for an alarming number of poisonings and deaths among teens.

**T**he misuse and abuse of drugs can lead to mental and emotional problems.

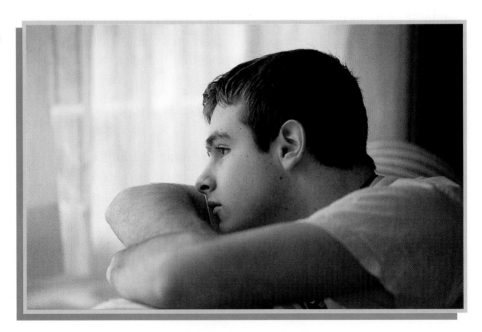

## DRUGS AND THEIR SIDE EFFECTS

| Amphetamines (Speed) | Cocaine (Coke, Snow) | Narcotics (Heroin: Smack) | Hallucinogens (LSD: Acid) (PCP: Angel dust) |
|---|---|---|---|
| • Brittle, broken-off hair | • Damage to lining of the nose | • Sexual problems | • Memory problems |
| • Bleeding gums | • Dilated pupils | • Shaking, muscle twitching | • Loss of judgment |
| • Weakened teeth that fall out | • Shaking, muscle twitching | • Slurred speech | • Fear, panic, terror |
| • Broken nails | • Vomiting | • Brain damage | • Depression, confusion, unpredictable or violent behavior |
| • Skin rashes | • Sweating | • Breathing difficulty | • Mood swings |
| • Anorexia nervosa (eating disorder that results in extreme thinness) | • Mood swings | • Heart problems | • Nausea, chills |
| • Addiction | • Seizures | • Collapsed veins, STIs, hepatitis, HIV/AIDS from needles | • Hallucinations |
| | • Liver damage | • Nausea, vomiting | • Elevated temperature, heart rate, blood pressure |
| | • Malnutrition | • Addiction | • Shaking |
| | • Heart attack | • Unconsciousness, death | • Coma |
| | • Stroke | | • Death |
| | • Addiction | | |
| | • Suicide, homicide | | |

GHB comes in many forms, liquid to powder to tablets. It also has many names, including *grievous bodily harm, G,* and *liquid Ecstasy.* The drug is often made in home laboratories.

The drug is abused mainly to get high. Some athletes, however, abuse it for its growth hormone-releasing effects, which build muscles. Undesired effects include trouble breathing, nausea, insomnia, anxiety, tremors, unconsciousness, coma, and death.

### Tranquilizers: The Calm Before the Storm

Doctors sometimes prescribe tranquilizers when their patients are feeling very nervous or troubled. Tranquilizers (TRAN·kwuh·ly·zurz) are *depressant drugs that make people feel tranquil, or calm.* The calm, however, lasts only as long as the drug is taken. Therefore, people can easily become addicted to, or hooked on, tranquilizers.

# Narcotics

**Narcotics** (nar·KAH·tiks) are *drugs sometimes used to relieve pain or bring about sleep.* Morphine and codeine are painkillers and may be prescribed by doctors. Illegal narcotics include heroin and opium. They come in powder and liquid form and are highly addictive. Drug users who inject narcotics are at risk for HIV, the virus that causes AIDS.

### No Heroes with Heroin

**Heroin** (HEHR·uh·win) is *a highly addictive narcotic* that can come in a white to dark brown powder. It can be snorted or smoked. It can also be injected into the bloodstream. This is called mainlining. Heroin can be deadly.

Heroin, also called *smack,* can give a powerful first rush, followed by a relaxed state or drowsiness. Then, however, it can lead to thinking problems, poor vision, trouble breathing, vomiting, constipation, increased need to urinate, itching or burning skin, sweats, low body temperature, brain damage, a desperate craving for more heroin, and death.

# Other Hallucinogens

In Lesson 7, you learned about marijuana, one popular drug that can cause hallucinations. Others to know about—and avoid—are PCP, ketamine, Ecstasy, and LSD.

### The Dangers of PCP

**PCP,** *a hallucinogen sometimes called "angel dust,"* can be a clear liquid, white powder, or pill. It changes a person's mood and affects perceptions. It can make a person feel terror or became violent. Muscle coordination is impaired, and the sensations of touch and pain are dulled. Time seems to pass slowly. PCP users can overdose or die because they lose their sense of time or space. PCP users have drowned in shallow water; they were so confused that they could not tell where they were or which direction was up.

### Ketamine

Ketamine is an anesthetic—a medicine meant to cause sleep during surgery. It is often used on animals. With the nicknames *special K, K,* and *vitamin K,* ketamine is a white powder, which is snorted, like cocaine. Users experience impaired attention, forgetfulness, high blood pressure, and sometimes death.

### The Agony of Ecstasy

One of the best-known designer drugs is the club drug *Ecstasy*, or *MDMA*. A combination stimulant and hallucinogen, Ecstasy may give the user a brief high. Its "lows" are far more dramatic. They include confusion, depression, and paranoia. Brain damage and increases in heart rate and blood pressure are other known effects. Using it even once can also lead to kidney failure, breathing problems, and death.

Herbal Ecstasy is *not* a safe alternative to Ecstasy. It, too, combines stimulant ingredients that can cause seizures, heart attack, stroke, and death.

### The Dangers of LSD

**LSD** is another *hallucinogen that is taken by mouth.* It can come in tablet form or in thin gelatin squares. Sometimes it is licked off blotter paper. LSD can cause side effects such as higher body temperature, sweating, paranoia, and intense terror. It can also cause *flashbacks,* serious drug effects long after the drug has been taken.

## Lesson 8 Review

Using complete sentences, answer the following questions on a sheet of paper.

### Reviewing Terms and Facts

1. **Recall** How are stimulants and depressants similar? How are they different?
2. **Vocabulary** What are *club drugs*? Name two and describe their negative health effects.

### Thinking Critically

3. **Synthesize** Choose a drug discussed in the lesson. Describe a specific emotional state or problem that might make a teen first want to use this substance to "solve" his or her problem. Describe how the drug might *worsen* instead of solve that problem and create new ones. Suggest better, chemical-free solutions.

### Applying Health Skills

4. **Advocacy** Choose one of the four classes of drugs discussed in the lesson. Based on what you have learned about the drug's effects, design a poster telling how you think a person who used this drug might look or act. Include an antidrug message on your poster.

# Refusal Skills and Responsible Decisions

**Describe two decisions you made this week that promoted your own health or the health of another person.**

## LEARN ABOUT...

- **how to deal with peer pressure.**
- **effective ways to use refusal skills against tobacco, alcohol, and other drugs.**
- **how to get involved in your community to help others choose a healthy, drug-free way of life.**

## VOCABULARY

- **peers**
- **manipulate**
- **refusal skills**
- **assertiveness**

Tobacco, alcohol, and other drugs are like thieves. They can rob teens of their looks, grades, talents, and health. Too often, they rob teens of their lives. By learning refusal skills, you can choose the healthy, happy route. You can choose to say yes to life—the only life you've got.

## Peer Influence: When the Pressure Is On

Your friends and classmates—your peers—no doubt play a key role in shaping the adult you will become. **Peers** are *people your own age who are similar to you in many ways.* Sometimes peers have a positive influence on you. Your peers may get you to join in worthwhile activities like team sports. They may show by their own example the importance of honesty and hard work.

At other times, though, this influence may not be so positive or healthy. Peer pressure to be "one of the gang" can also lead teens to use tobacco, alcohol, and other drugs.

### Friendly Fire

The toughest kind of peer pressure to resist is when a friend or group of friends is doing the pressuring. In fact, the majority of teens who use substances say that they would not have started if their friends or peers had not encouraged them to do so.

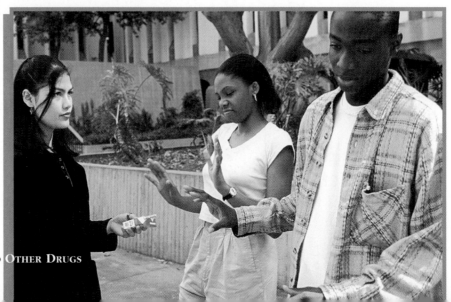

**P**racticing refusal skills is important. *Why is it important?*

Peers can try to **manipulate** (muh·NIP·yuh·layt) you. They try to *influence you in an indirect, unfair, or deceitful way.* Remember this: True friends don't try to control each other. They respect one's right to say no and to disagree. They don't act hurt or angry if you feel strongly about something or if you are sticking up for the values you hold dear.

## Effective Refusal Skills

How other people behave toward you and around you is usually beyond your control. However, *you* have the power over your own decisions. When peers pressure you to use tobacco, alcohol, or other drugs, say no. Faced with real-life pressures, though, you may have to practice using your refusal skills. **Refusal skills** are *strategies that help you say no effectively.* Some strategies work better than others for different people in different situations. However, they all work best when you are sticking up for what you believe.

Saying no effectively is partly a matter of style—your body language and the attitude you show. Speak in a firm voice with your head and shoulders up. This will tell the other person that you mean what you say. This is **assertiveness**, *showing that you will stand up for your own rights but that you are respectful of the rights of others.* This makes it easier to stand your ground.

## Be Prepared

It is important to practice refusal skills in advance. Trouble often happens when you least expect it, so it is best to be prepared. Take Tom's situation, for example. One day after school, some older teens invite him to join their skateboarding club. Tom is so pleased to be included that he accepts when they offer him a cigarette to "make it official." Soon, he finds himself smoking whenever he hangs out with his new friends. He even begins craving cigarettes at other times. Tom could have avoided becoming addicted if he had practiced refusal skills and said no when he was offered that first cigarette.

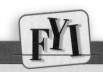

### Having No-How

Refusal skills are really a matter of "no-how": knowing how to say no. The following tips may help:

- Take your time. Stall if you have to in order to collect your thoughts.
- State how you feel. Be direct. Keep your statements short.
- Use "I," not "You," messages. Don't blame or name-call.
- Stand up straight and use direct eye contact. Speak in a firm voice.
- Don't apologize for your values.
- Suggest more health-ful alternatives.
- Leave if you have to. Just walk away.

**T**here are many ways of saying no. *Which do you think would be most effective for you?*

# Three Real Choices

When it comes to tobacco, alcohol, and other drugs, there are only three healthy choices:

1. If you have never used them, decide right now that you will *never* start. Build a strong support system to help you stay substance free.

2. If you have experimented with these substances, decide right now not to do it again. Remember, trouble creeps up on teens who experiment with substances.

3. If you think you may be in real trouble with substance abuse, get help right away. Talk to a school counselor, school nurse, or trusted adult; or call one of the organizations discussed in this booklet and someone will tell you how and where to get the help you need. Do it *now!*

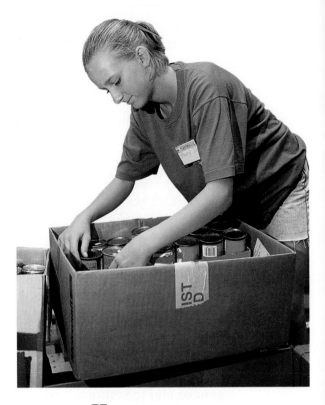

**H**elping out in your community is one healthful alternative to drugs. *Name some other healthful alternatives.*

## Lesson 9 Review

Using complete sentences, answer the following questions on a sheet of paper.

### Reviewing Terms and Facts

1. **Vocabulary** What are *refusal skills*?
2. **Recall** Describe how trouble might creep up on a teen who smokes, drinks, or uses other drugs without him or her realizing it right away.

### Thinking Critically

3. **Synthesize** Andy lives with his mom and his older brother, Jim, who is in high school. His dad passed away, and Jim works part-time to help pay the bills. Sometimes Jim goes out and uses drugs with his friends. In what ways might Jim's drug use affect his family, job, and community?

### Applying Health Skills

4. **Goal Setting** Make a time line of your life using a long strip of paper (such as computer paper). Divide the time line into four sections: ages 12–15, ages 16–18, ages 19–21, and ages 22–25. Write down one or two goals for each period. In a separate section, write down the ways that using alcohol or drugs might get in the way of achieving these goals.

# Glossary

 **A**

**Abuse** Using drugs in ways that are unhealthy or illegal. *(page 1)*

**Addicted** Dependent on a drug. *(page 3)*

**Addiction** Condition in which a person is psychologically or physically dependent on a chemical substance. *(page 15)*

**Alcoholism** A physical and mental addiction to alcohol. *(page 15)*

**Anabolic steroids** Synthetic forms of the male hormone testosterone. *(page 29)*

**Assertiveness** Showing that you will stand up for your own rights but that you are respectful of the rights of others. *(page 37)*

 **B**

**BAC** The amount of alcohol in the blood. *(page 12)*

**Binge drinking** Drinking four or five or more drinks in a short period of time. *(page 24)*

 **C**

**Carbon monoxide** A poisonous gas that cannot be seen or smelled. *(page 21)*

**Cells** Tiny, complex units that make up all plants and animals. *(page 5)*

**Cirrhosis** Destruction of cells and scarring of liver tissues. *(page 6)*

**Club drugs** Illegal substances that got their start at adult clubs. *(page 31)*

**Crack** A crystallized form of cocaine that can be smoked. *(page 31)*

 **D**

**Dehydration** The loss of important body fluids. *(page 24)*

**Depressant** A drug that can slow down the activity of the brain and nervous system. *(pages 22, 32)*

**Drug Free Zone** A 1,000-yard distance around a school. *(page 12)*

**Drugs** Substances other than food that you take into your body and that change the way your mind and body work. *(page 1)*

 **E**

**Endurance** The ability to keep your energy level up. *(page 7)*

**Ethanol** A type of alcohol that is produced naturally when the sugars from fruits, grains, or vegetables are fermented with yeast. *(page 22)*

 **G**

**Gateway drugs** Drugs that can lead to using other drugs. *(page 3)*

 **H**

**Hallucinogen** A drug that creates imaginary images or distorts real ones in the user's mind. *(page 26)*

**Heroin** Highly addictive narcotic. *(page 34)*

**Hormones** Substances in your body that direct certain aspects of growth and development. *(page 7)*

 **I**

**Inhalant** Vapors of chemicals that are sniffed or inhaled to get a "high." *(page 28)*

**Insecticides** Chemicals used to kill insects. *(page 20)*

 **L**

**LSD** Hallucinogen that is taken by mouth. *(page 35)*

 **M**

**Manipulate** Influence in an indirect, unfair, or deceitful way. *(page 37)*

**Marijuana** Made from the dried leaves and flower of the hemp plant, cannabis. *(page 26)*

**Medicine** Legal drug used to cure diseases or stop pain. *(page 1)*

**Metabolism** Process by which the body turns food into energy. *(page 23)*

**Minors** People under the age of adult rights and responsibilities. *(page 11)*

**Misuse** Taking or using medicine in a way that is not intended. *(page 1)*

**Motor skills** Control of your muscles and physical coordination. *(page 6)*

# Glossary

**Narcotics** Drugs sometimes used to relieve pain or bring about sleep. *(page 34)*

**Nicotine** The substance in tobacco that causes its drug effects. *(page 20)*

**Overdose** Taking more of a drug than a body can stand. *(page 3)*

**Paranoia** A feeling that others are out to get them. *(page 26)*

**PCP** A hallucinogen sometimes called "angel dust." *(page 34)*

**Peers** People your own age who are similar to you in many ways. *(page 36)*

**Possess** To have with you or on you. *(page 11)*

**Probation** A set period of time during which an offender must check in regularly with a court officer. *(page 10)*

**Reflexes** The body's natural muscle reactions. *(page 7)*

**Refusal skills** Strategies that help you say no effectively. *(page 37)*

**Secondhand smoke** Smoke that you inhale by being near someone who is smoking. *(page 21)*

**Smokeless tobacco** Dried, ground-up tobacco leaves. *(page 18)*

**Snuff** Processed wet or dry tobacco powder. *(page 19)*

**Sobriety checkpoints** Places where police officers check drivers for drugs and alcohol. *(page 12)*

**Stimulant** Drug that speeds up heart and breathing rate and raises blood pressure. *(pages 20, 30)*

**Tar** Dark, sticky liquid made when tobacco burns. *(page 20)*

**Tolerance** The need for more of a substance to get the same effect. *(page 15)*

**Toxic** Poisonous. *(page 24)*

**Tranquilizers** Depressant drugs. *(page 33)*

**Ulcers** Open sores in the stomach lining. *(page 25)*

**Withdrawal** A series of painful physical and mental symptoms associated with recovery from a drug. *(page 15)*

# Glosario

**Abuse/Abuso** Usar drogas de manera no saludable o ilegal. *(página 1)*

**Addicted/Adicto** Dependiente de una droga. *(página 3)*

**Addiction/Adicción** Condición en la cual una persona depende fisiológica o físicamente de una sustancia química. *(página 15)*

**Alcoholism/Alcoholismo** Adicción física y mental al alcohol. *(página 15)*

**Anabolic Steroids/Esteroides anabólicos** Formas sintéticas de la hormona masculina testosterona. *(página 29)*

**Assertiveness/Seguridad propia** Mostrar que se defienden los derechos propios, pero se respetan los derechos de otros. *(página 37)*

**BAC/Contenido alcohólico de la sangre** Cantidad de alcohol en la sangre. *(página 12)*

**Binge drinking/Tomar en parranda** Ingerir cuatro, cinco o más tragos en un período corto de tiempo. *(página 24)*

**Carbon monoxide/Monóxido de carbono** Gas venenoso que no se ve o se huele. *(página 21)*

**Cells/Células** Unidades pequeñas complejas que forman las plantas y los animales. *(página 5)*

**Cirrhosis/Cirrosis** Destrucción de células y icatrices de los tejidos del hígado. *(página 6)*

**Club drugs/Drogas sociales** Sustancias ilegales que comienzan a usarse en clubes de adultos. *(página 31)*

**Crack/Crack** Forma cristalizada de la cocaína que se puede fumar. *(página 31)*

**Dehydration/Deshidratación** Pérdida de fluidos importantes del cuerpo. *(página 24)*

**Depressant/Sedativo** Droga que aminora la actividad del cerebro y el sistema nervioso. *(páginas 22, 32)*

**Drug Free Zone/Zona protegida antidroga** 1,000 yardas de distancia alrededor de una escuela. *(página 12)*

**Drugs/Drogas** Sustancias que no son alimentos que se pueden introducir al cuerpo y cambian la manera en que funcionan la mente y el cuerpo. *(página 1)*

**Endurance/Resistencia** Habilidad de mantener el nivel de energía alto. *(página 7)*

**Ethanol/Etanol** Tipo de alcohol que se produce naturalmente cuando se fermentan con levadura los azúcares de las frutas, los granos o los vegetales. *(página 22)*

**Gateway drugs/Drogas de enlace** Drogas que pueden conducir al uso de otras drogas. *(página 3)*

**Hallucinogen/Alucinógenos** Droga que crea imágenes imaginarias o distorsionan las reales en la mente de quien la usa. *(página 26)*

**Heroin/Heroína** Narcótico sumamente aditivo. *(página 34)*

**Hormones/Hormonas** Sustancias en el cuerpo que dirigen ciertos aspectos del crecimiento y desarrollo. *(página 7)*

**Inhalant/Inhalante** Vapores de sustancias químicas que se huelen o inhalan para endrogarse. *(página 28)*

**Insecticides/Insecticidas** Sustancias químicas que se usan para matar insectos. *(página 20)*

**LSD/LSD** Alucinógeno que se ingiere oralmente. *(página 35)*

**Manipulate/Manipular** Influencia de forma indirecta, injusta o engañosa. *(página 37)*

**Marijuana/Marihuana** Hecha de hojas y flores secas de la planta de cáñamo índico, cannabis indico. *(página 26)*

**Medicine/Medicina** Droga legal usada para curar enfermedades o suprimir el dolor. *(página 1)*

# Glosario

**Metabolism/Metabolismo** Proceso por el cual el cuerpo convierte los alimentos en energía. *(página 23)*

**Minors/Menores de edad** Personas no adultas sin los derechos y las responsabilidades de éstas. *(página 11)*

**Misuse/Mal uso** Tomar o usar medicina de forma no indicada. *(página 1)*

**Motor skills/Destrezas motoras** Control de los músculos y coordinación física. *(página 6)*

**Narcotics/Narcóticos** Drogas que se usan algunas veces para aliviar el dolor o dormir. *(página 34)*

**Nicotine/Nicotina** La sustancia en el tabaco que causa efectos aditivos. *(página 20)*

**Overdose/Sobredosis** Tomar más de una droga de la que el cuerpo puede tolerar. *(página 3)*

**Paranoia/Paranoia** Sentimiento de que otros lo persiguen. *(página 26)*

**PCP/PCP** Alucinógeno a veces llamado "polvo de ángel." *(página 34)*

**Peers/Compañeros** Personas de tu edad que se parecen a ti en muchas maneras. *(página 36)*

**Posses/Poseer** Tener con uno o en uno. *(página 11)*

**Probation/Período de prueba** Un período de tiempo establecido durante el cual un ofensor debe reportarse regularmente ante un oficial del tribunal. *(página 10)*

**Reflexes/Reflejos** Las reacciones naturales de los músculos del cuerpo. *(página 7)*

**Refusal skills/Destrezas de negación** Estrategias que ayudan a decir no efecvtivamente. *(página 37)*

**Secondhand smoke/Humo de segunda mano** Humo que se inhala al estar cerca de alguien que fuma. *(página 21)*

**Smokeless tobacco/Tabaco sin humo** Hojas de tabaco secas molidas. *(página 18)*

**Snuff/Oler** Polvo procesado de tabaco mojado o seco. *(página 19)*

**Sobriety checkpoints/Puntos de inspección de sobriedad** Lugares donde la policía inspecciona la influencia de drogas y alcohol en conductores. *(página 12)*

**Stimulant/Estimulantes** Droga que acelera los latidos del corazón y la respiración y eleva la presión arterial. *(páginas 20, 30)*

**Tar/Alquitrán** Líquido oscuro y pegagoso producido por el tabaco al quemarse. *(página 20)*

**Tolerance/Tolerancia** Más cantidad de la sustancia para obtener el mismo efecto. *(página 15)*

**Toxic/Tóxico** Veneno. *(página 24)*

**Tranquilizers/Tranquilizantes** Drogas sedativas. *(página 33)*

**Ulcers/Úlceras** Llagas abiertas en las paredes del estómago. *(página 25)*

**Withdrawal/Aislamiento** Serie de síntomas físicos y mentales asociados con la recuperación de una droga. *(página 15)*

# Index

Note: Page numbers in *italics* refer to art and marginal features.

# Index